Forget Obama Trump Ignored
Volume One

HEALTH CARE!

How to lower costs
and
restore our collective sanity

2nd Edition

by

Brian J. Dixon M.D.

For information about the coming renaissance, visit

www.togetherforward.org

dedicated to Momma

Foreword

I get it. We've all been there – another great idea from someone that we don't know (or trust) encouraging us to jump on their bandwagon to idiocracy. Sometimes it's from the rich politician suggesting legislation with consequences completely disconnected from their lavish lifestyle. Other times it's from the dreamer whose ideas are so big and truly wonderful that you know there is no hope for it ever changing.

Needless to say, when Brian first shared his plan to change healthcare, I smiled, nodded, and rolled my eyes (internally). But after years of "hmmm" moments, and as much as it pains me to get my hopes up, his plan is ingenious and **may actually work**.

Brian and I know one another through running our own private practices in mental health. Though we share similar views in our passion for quality patient care, our financial models of practice are night and day. His psychiatry practice works on a direct pay basis (no insurance), while my group therapy practice accepts almost every insurance plan available. As a licensed clinical social worker, foster/adoptive mom of five kids, and a certified bleeding heart, my goal is to make services as affordable and accessible as possible to all individuals in our community. Yet, the longer I practice, the more our current healthcare system makes this nearly impossible. I won't get into the nitty-gritty, but I think Brian's book does a fabulous job outlining why doctors and therapists are discarding their insurance contracts.

The real reason why I believe his plan works? I'm accidentally living it. I have been uninsured for the past four or so years. When I first stepped into the world of self-employment, I paid privately for insurance – nearly $500.00 per MONTH. That lasted a good six to eight months before I realized I couldn't afford the monthly premium, especially when I hadn't even used the insurance for any reason. I went another three years of being a cash pay client (no insurance, no catastrophic coverage, nada). *Sadly, the fines to my income for not having health insurance were still less than the premiums I would have paid for an insurance I never used* [remember, poor social worker here]. Only recently have I joined a type of health co-op which I consider similar to catastrophic coverage.

I am cheap, but I value my health. I want to live a long time for my kiddos. That said, Brian's plan encourages accountability and resourcefulness. As someone who is professionally reaping the negative consequences of our current healthcare system alongside the personal benefits of living this model, I say with confidence that his idea works. Here's my challenge to you: Open your eyes to the possibilities of what could be. Brian tells everyone to "stay woke." Here's your first guide. Trust me, it's a fun ride on what we thought was a beaten topic.

- Anastasia "Stas" Taylor, MSSW, LCSW

Preface

As a child psychiatrist and behavior therapist, my patients don't tend to lie on the couch and pontificate. So, I designed this book much like I would one of my private sessions. You ask me common questions about healthcare reform and I tell you the ugly truth. Lucky for you, I'll give you the actual answer to the problem (my patients have to find their own, and fortunately most of them do).

There is a ridiculous amount written about why our healthcare system is jacked up. When you go "huh?", be sure to check out the endnotes for details.

- Brian J Dixon MD

Second Edition Notes
Time flies. Reforming healthcare finance is daunting, but I can think of nothing else I'd rather do. Since the launch of the first edition, I've talked to hundreds of stakeholders in the form of patients and physicians. I've seen frustration from all sides and commiserated with their disappointment that a "solution" hasn't been found.

This revised second edition expounds on ideas introduced in the first book and offers perspective on new areas like residency and current "solutions." The medical and financial landscape of healthcare is changing quickly, and I hope you'll find the added chapters useful. It's time for big discussions about uncomfortable topics, including the role of nurse practitioners, physician suicide, and the corporatization of medicine.

Chapters 15 through 22 are all new material (and not for the faint of heart.) You ask tough questions and I give hard and honest answers. We may not always agree, but believe this: The best healthcare solution revolves around the patient-physician relationship.
                                        -BJD

Introduction to Reading this Book

Instead of encouraging you to skip the foreplay and head straight to the climax, I put the climax front and center for you in Chapter One. You're welcome.

We know our healthcare finance system is horrible, thus there's no need to read any other chapter. However, I think you should (since I spent time writing it), and you may learn a thing or two that compels you to change our society, our minds, our lives. Each chapter is written as a conversation, with most drawn from real-life discussions with patients, doctors, administrators, and government officials over the last five years.

Chapter 0.5, however, is required. Consider it a polite "intervention," so that you know your role in creating our current healthcare boondoggle and can take responsibility for your skewed views before committing to fix it.

If you're not ready to change, close this book and keep whining about the cost of care to people who can't fix it (politicians, your doctor, your family, your friends.) Like Smokey the Medical Bear says, "Only YOU can fix healthcare financing."

Your questions and comments are in **bold**; I respond in kind. Ain't I nice?

TABLE OF CONTENTS

<u>Chapter 0.5</u>

Whose fault is it?
Americans love to assign blame. Fortunately for us, there's a lot of blame to go around when it comes to healthcare. It's mostly your fault (yes you, the reader) but "all have sinned and fallen short of the glory." Let's detail the other culprits first and we'll get to you soon enough. Here we go:

- Doctors
- Health Insurance Companies
- Government
- Hospitals
- Drug Companies
- "Privacy"
- You

What did Doctors do?
We created the American Medical Association (AMA) to protect physicians' market share. In its zeal to protect the profession, the AMA agreed to financial models that created devastating unintended consequences.

In her book, *Ensuring America's Health*, Dr. Christy Ford Chapin shows how doctors of the AMA put into motion the broken financial system we have today. I won't belabor the point (read her book—it's terrific).

It took me a while to realize we don't have a healthcare quality issue. Most doctors are, in fact, phenomenal men and women who sacrifice decades and amass huge debts to improve other people's health. What we have is a HEALTHCARE FINANCE issue. Money (business, management, finance) is not the physician's speciality. When we relinquished our role as healthcare administrators, we put it into the hands of (mostly) men who would do anything for a buck. And they did. They made lots of bucks and they gave you none.

Was it Health Insurance Companies?
First and foremost, let's be clear: Health insurance companies are not evil. They're companies. Their goal is to make money for their shareholders. In and of itself, this is not a bad thing.

Unfortunately, their desire to turn a profit often conflicts with being decent human beings.

What about the Government?
The government's role is to "...provide for the common defence, promote the general Welfare, and secure the Blessings of Liberty to ourselves and our

Posterity...." Oftentimes, that means taking a little and stretching it out as "fairly" as possible.

The government is us. We are the government. When we decided to build a union and fight for a union, we agreed to combine resources and share for the common good. But we took it too far when it came to healthcare finance. After Americans wanted more healthcare on their own terms and doctors acquiesced to colluding with insurance companies, the government kicked into high gear by building a *privileged structure on a universal right.* Clean air, water, and preventative public care are all rights. Having the newest medical device *when* you want it but on someone *else's* dime is not.

And Hospitals?
People forget that hospitals are businesses in competition with each other. They want to turn a tidy profit and have found lots of ways to shroud this fact in plain view.

I'm not sure how a for-profit business like a hospital was able to get "nonprofit" status, but that's a subject for a later chapter. Hospitals exacerbate healthcare financial woes *because they hide their price lists.*

I'm sure those pesky Drug Companies are in on it too, right?
Drug companies, another for-profit entity in the healthcare arena, take well-meaning scientific

discoveries, monetize them, and play on our need for wellness and non-death.

They don't care about your health. I know it sounds like a bitter pill to swallow but, honestly, the sooner we accept this truth the better off we'll be. When Merck jacked up the price of their EpiPen, they had every right to do so. And they deserved all the repercussions.

How is HIPAA an issue?

Americans love their privacy as much as they love their liberty. In a world of increased information sharing, well-meaning intentions turn funky, fast.

Walled-off communication actually blocks your healthcare providers from knowing your full history. This leads to repetition of exams, which wastes time, and lab test duplication, which wastes money. Multiply that times 100 million, and you get my drift.

YOU!

Yes, reader of this awesome book—YOU are driving up the cost of your own care through both your expectations and your investments. If you own stock in an index fund that includes any health insurance company, then you're at fault. *If you've ever wanted manscanning* (i.e. "doc, I feel bad, run every test and scan you can think of"), *then you've enabled the problem in some form or fashion.*

So, what do we do?

Rest easy, my fellow American. With the help of your friendly, health-reform-savvy "shrink by proxy," you can fix this.

Chapter 1: Shrink's Fix – Part 1

What's the right question?
The first step in fixing anything is to ask the right question. We've spent decades trying to figure this one out:

"How do we get more people insured?"

I am an unabashed lover of President Barack Obama. But when he tried to improve healthcare (a noble goal, to be sure), he doubled down on a faulty premise built on a faulty question. The result: a faulty answer.

To fix this correctly, let's start with a better question:

"How do we change market forces to tilt healthcare financing in the patients' favor?"

Let's start with recognizing that the practice of

American healthcare isn't the issue. I personally have yet to meet a physician whose primary goal is to make money. We love caring for patients. In our fallible humanity, physicians sacrifice a lot of time, energy, and money to become expert educated guessers with hopes of alleviating another's suffering. Cost is an afterthought in most medical encounters, so ensuring we have a transparent financial structure is more important now than ever.

Multiplying a risky proposition (insurance) and an educated guess (healthcare) just screws shit up. So, instead of trying to build a financial system based on absolutes (which don't exist), let's instead build a financial system where humans are in control of paying for the educated guesses they want and need.

Okay, so how do we fix it then?
First, get rid of the notion that you are powerless and that "the government" is out to hurt us. YOU ARE THE GOVERNMENT!!! (*...*if you voted*. If you didn't vote, then stop reading, go register, and come back. I'll wait...*).

Only registered voters may continue:

You are powerful, and for this idea to work, you must own your shit, hold yourself accountable, and build a society of people you trust to own their own shit too.

We've laid the foundation; now let's get down to brass tacks:

Step One
Create 50 nonprofit statewide health companies, one for each state. Every citizen 18+ is a shareholder.

Step Two
The shareholders elect a Board of Directors, 60 percent of whom must be licensed health professionals (e.g. physicians, nurses, dentists, therapists, acupuncturists, etc.).

Step Three
The Board of Directors establishes the state chargemaster. This will be the standard "price guide" for all diagnoses used by providers in the state. The chargemaster divides visits into "preventative" and "sick" categories.

Step Four
The Board of Directors establishes the General Health Fee. This is the fee that every person pays yearly into the General Health Fund for the state. This fund pays for preventative visits for all citizens, as well as healthcare costs for diagnoses unrelated to personal lifestyle choices.

Step Five
The Board of Directors of all states vote on and choose one universal electronic medical record. While the health record will be a commercially

available product, it will be backed by the cybersecurity strength of the federal government.

Step Six

The Board of Directors, as a private company, will use market forces to leverage down the cost of medications/medical devices because they can buy their meds/devices in bulk from wherever they want. (Personally, I recommend the United Kingdom and Canada for medications and devices. American companies sell the exact same meds under a different name for a fraction of the cost. Since Brits and Canadians aren't dropping dead on a daily basis, they must be doing something right).

What's a "preventative visit"?

Paying one's health fee every year entitles that person to a preventative visit composed of:

- Medical exam (pap smears, mammograms, prostate exams, etc.)
- Mental health screening with a mental health professional
- Dental visit (x-rays and cleanings)
- Vision care (corrective lenses)
- Basic labs
- Up to three months of medications

Alright, what's a "sick visit"?

A "sick visit" is anything that happens outside of a preventative visit. Sometimes this is emergency care, urgent care, or any other time you'd choose to go see a doctor. If the diagnosis rendered is unrelated to lifestyle choices, you'd be able to get reimbursed for the cost of that diagnosis (as listed on your state's chargemaster).

Why do you care?
Because I believe.

Because I believe in *Pollyanna*.

Because I believe people are capable of great compassion.

Because I believe endless creativity begins when we are fed, safe, educated, and cared for.

Because I believe American ingenuity makes us a unique force in the world (and the galaxy).

Because I believe it's stupid to have business people and politicians overrule your healthcare provider.

Because I believe we are killing ourselves by allowing the healthcare finance system to metastasize.

Seriously, won't you make a ton of money in the current system?
Technically, yes. My private practice model is pretty lucrative. But I don't see patients for the money. I love helping people to feel better and to live their best lives.

I was a recipient of government assistance when I was younger (the colorful food stamps were all the rage back then), and for that reason, I am compelled to build a better system. Better systems lead to better societies and, eventually, better starships (like the Enterprise-D).

Um...aren't you afraid someone's gonna hurt you for this radical idea?
I've had multiple psychiatrist friends encourage me to hire armed protection. So, yeah, I'm sure this idea will piss off lots of rich folks who own, manage, or benefit from our skewed healthcare finance system.

Some will say, "Well, this is just a redistribution of wealth." They'd be correct. Disparity must exist for an economy to function. But a large disparity grinds the whole damn thing to a halt because there's no way for the "have nots" to ever "have" since the "haves" essentially "have it all."

And what do you call this?
I'm terrible at marketing (because I'm a trained physician, not a marketer), but I like the term **PSYCH: P**ractical **S**olutions **Y**ielding **C**omprehensive **H**ealthcare. I think it has a great ring to it. But you can refer to it as "that crazy idea that psychiatrist had" and I'm sure it'll suffice for now.

I have more questions about your plan!!!

Great! Visit Chapters 9 through 13 for more discussion. Also, Chapters 2 to 8 expose the major players contributing to the quagmire.

And finally, I spent a cool five grand on an explainer video, so go watch it: www.changhealth.today.

Chapter 2: Health Insurance

Why is health insurance so expensive?
Because insurance companies make it that way.

Contrary to popular belief, companies make up their own pricing. Sure, they use actuaries and "market analysis" to compare the pricing of their competitors, but the price of something comes down to a single person/committee majority vote. So when Big Insurance raises your premiums, it's because they want to.

It really IS that simple.

How do we lower the cost of health insurance?
Vote with your wallet.

Theoretically, in our capitalistic system, if everyone got fed up with commercial insurance, they would simply switch. The loss of profit and market share would "teach" that company to change (if they wanted to stay in existence). It's simple supply and demand.

Unfortunately, because of the Affordable Care Act, we're forced to purchase a commercial product whose cost we can't control. In other words, we can't leverage the power of our pocketbook because we're forced to buy a product where there are only a few players to choose from (not unlike the airline industry).

So then why do we do prior authorizations?
When I look at "stupid" processes in American healthcare, this is probably the stupidest.

Prior authorizations were meant to ensure the prescribed treatment from the physician was appropriate for the patient. Stupid. If I write a prescription, obviously I think my patient should have it. The fact that I, an educated and licensed physician, has to take time to beg an insurance company full of mathematicians to approve a treatment I've already approved of is just plain stupid.

So, why do insurance companies make you do them?

Because it saves greedy insurance companies money. Not you. Let's walk through it:

You (the patient) pay a monthly premium to access a pool of medical providers with whom the insurance company contracts. *The insurance company has a vested interest in not paying back the money you gave them*, thereby earning them a "profit" to pay their shareholders. Insurance companies have any number of ways to keep from paying out, and prior authorizations are an added "hurdle" that some patients and doctors don't want to deal with. The result is that the patient will either drop the treatment or use a different treatment they know both of which are likely more affordable to the insurance company.

In and of itself, prior authorizations are not a bad idea for the insurance company since it is designed to make a profit. But when it conflicts with appropriate patient care, that's a problem.

Insurance companies recognize how crappy this is, so, on the whole, they try to allow most "usual and customary" treatments (i.e. costs and treatments a reasonable person thinks would be fair). Unfortunately, the stupid hurdles are far more common than the "reasonable" hurdles.

For example, I had a young patient with autism who did really well on a brand name medicine we'll call "Ability." Ability costs a lot of money (see Chapter 6), and though there is a generic version, there's something about brand name Ability that works really well for this kiddo. His ideal dose was 10mg. Oddly enough, he didn't do well with one tablet of the 10mg, but with two tablets of the 5mg, he was amazing. You'd think it would be an easy prescription request.

Sadly, you 'd be wrong. Sixty tablets of Ability 5mg actually cost twice as much as 30 tablets of Ability 10mg. Physicians and patients have to call, beg, and waste hours of our time on the phone to get this treatment authorized. How does any of that benefit patient care?

It doesn't. There's no other way to put it, prior authorizations suck.

And the same is true for "out of network"?
Yup!

"In network" and "out of network" are additional roadblocks that insurance companies created to keep their money. Since insurance is so commonplace for primary care and medical subspecialties, medical providers in those specialties are super pressured to be on an insurance panel.

The medical providers (e.g., doctors, hospitals, pharmacies) that are "in-network," have been locked by the insurance company into accepting a certain amount of payment from them. You pay your predetermined copay and, on the back end, the insurance company sends a check to the doctor *if* they've filled out *all* the correct forms. Every medical condition has a "code", and insurance companies change whatever codes they like and don't like all the time without even notifying physicians. This leads to regular miscoding, which leads to payment denials, payment delays, stressed out physician office staff, and very bitter physicians.

Insurance companies loathe paying psychiatrists what they're worth, so more of us are opting to be "out of network." With the addiction and mental health issues in America today, imagine the consequences.

Why doesn't [insert doctor's name] take my insurance?

Because doctors don't make money by contracting with insurance companies.

When a physician enters into a contract with an insurance company, they are essentially agreeing to take a set amount of money in exchange for having "access" to an insurance company's panel of patients.

By law, we as physicians are not allowed to charge different prices to different people (more on that later). Contracts that are percentage-based, drive up the cost. For example, if BlueCross is willing to pay me 50 percent of charges, then I'm going to charge as much as possible. The kicker: Once I've locked in my rates, then I have to charge direct paying patients the same thing. It's a hidden glitch in the law because insurance companies (rightfully) don't want to be price gouged. The result: Direct paying people get gouged instead.

But I benefit from the ACA and I hate Obamacare!
face palm

The Affordable Care Act (ACA) and "Obamacare" (OC) are the exact same thing. The ACA is a law establishing that every person must have health insurance. On its face, it sounds both fair and progressive. But behind the scenes, it all falls apart because all health insurance is a private product that a company sells to you.

The devil is in the details of the terms and conditions of that product. Before the ACA/OC, health insurance plans could have lots of holes in them. For example, they wouldn't cover mental health. This was perfectly fine for people who didn't have mental health concerns and were fine with their holey plans and the price they were paying.

But what happened when that person subsequently had a mental health issue? They then discovered they had no coverage and, because costs are opaque in our system, the costs they had to pay were astronomical. They rightfully howled at their employers and Congresspeople. But instead of fixing the basic premise of our flawed financial system, we all doubled down on forcing insurance companies to "cover" more things. When insurance companies "cover" more conditions, they pay out more money, their revenue drops, and they say "screw it—we're either going to stop selling these products or we're gonna charge you more!"

Hence, insurance premiums go up each year and people get angrier about "Obamacare."

Yes, but none of this was bad until Obama came along!
double face palm

Healthcare finance has been an issue for decades. Different politicians have tried different approaches (Hillary Clinton in the 1990s and Mitt Romney as governor of Massachusetts in the 2000s), but each comes up short because they build well-meaning systems on a broken premise.

What about "reinsurance"?
triple face palm (which requires someone else to hit me upside the head)

Full disclaimer: I think the concept of reinsurance is so dumb I'm shaking in anger as I write this.

Reinsurance is the federal government giving health insurance companies money when the health insurance companies feel they've paid out too much money to care for people with ACA/OC health plans. I shit you not.

In your plan, will I need insurance?

Nope. Insurance will be optional and you'll be able to decide what level of catastrophic insurance you want to carry.

For example, smoking cigarettes is your constitutional right. You know it's unhealthy so you buy insurance for the recurrent bronchitis flare-ups and pneumonia that require expensive intensive care. And the opposite is true: If you choose to eat a vegan diet, carry an advanced directive, and workout, you can fearlessly go without catastrophic care insurance and tax penalties.

But what if you're in an accident?
Now that you won't have to buy health insurance, you can buy accident insurance instead, which should cover you according to auto/house/property liability insurance rules.

And remember: In my plan, if it's not your fault, your costs will be covered according to your state's chargemaster for "conditions unrelated to lifestyle choices." A non-smoking woman diagnosed with gene positive breast cancer will have more treatment costs reimbursed than her similar peer who smokes (Flip to Chapter 13 for more discussion).

Chapter 3: The Government

Why blame the government?
Technically, the government is us (the people), so our failing healthcare system is largely our own fault (see Chapter 8).

But since we've been doing such a great job of projecting our shortcomings onto one another for the last half-century, let's tackle the "government" issue as if it's an entity apart from us.

We've agreed to make sacrifices to ensure our society works based on fairness. When we sense unfairness (like in healthcare), it threatens our social commitment to one another.

But seriously, why can't Congress fix this?
Because they're not qualified nor are they supposed to.

Take a moment and read the Constitution (https://www.archives.gov/founding-docs/constitution-transcript).

I'll wait.

Notice that there's no mention of healthcare? That's because those rights and responsibilities fell to the individual to manage.

The Constitution gives Congress the power to make laws that don't violate the Constitution. So, Congress passed legislation to try and help. I suggest that the current legislation is actually causing more harm than good and needs to be repealed. Medicare was the first mistake. Congress followed with "fixes" for a broken system that only exacerbated the misunderstanding of how healthcare financing should work.

Is healthcare a privilege or a right?
While I'm not a constitutional scholar, I would contend that basic preventative care is a right while all sick care is a privilege.

The Preamble of the Constitution states: "We the People of the United States, in order to form a more perfect Union, establish Justice, insure domestic Tranquility, provide for the common defence, promote the general Welfare, and secure the Blessings of Liberty to ourselves and our Posterity, do ordain and establish this Constitution for the United States of America."

I think the federal government's role to "insure domestic Tranquility...promote the general Welfare" means that we provide public health to the masses. We've done that: vaccinations, well-trained and accountable physicians, and freely accessible media/information outlets. With the invention of the Internet, any educated citizen can do a more than reasonable job of caring for themselves.

However, having the latest CT scan, newest medication, and medical "on-call" services isn't a right. That's a privilege. As a society, we've established that privileges must be paid for. Fortunately, we're learning that "new" isn't always "better", and that a good verbal history coupled with some older medications can be just as effective as new devices with all the bells and whistles.

So, Medicare is bad then, right?
Any system built on health insurance is bad because "We the People" can't directly control the cost of a private product. Medicare is no exception. When the government got into the "health insurance" business, they essentially made a private product, priced that product, and then took away the ability for the individual citizen and their doctors to adjust it.

<u>Chapter 4: Physicians</u>

Wait, doctors caused this?

Sorta. During her search to find historical data on
why our healthcare system is so warped, Dr. Christy
Ford Chapin made some startling revelations:

Doctors were hell-bent on protecting their
profession from outside snake oil salesmen (a noble
goal) but went about it by building on top of
commercial insurance (a terrible idea). The results
were decades of unintended consequences, but it
made great business sense in their time.

What were these unintended consequences?

For example, when the government and the AMA
agreed to work together on Medicare, they created a
panel composed of the heads of all medical specialty
boards. Someone (or multiple someones) in that
group decided that physical procedures should be
reimbursed at a higher rate than non-procedures.

By definition, procedures are physically invasive
actions: suturing, removing moles, and giving IV

medicines. Diabetes education, counseling, and using a stethoscope are not. For some reason, those physicians deemed procedures more valuable than non-procedures.

This singular decision still reverberates today because *many doctors avoid low-paying fields* (like primary care and psychiatry) for higher paying fields (surgery and surgical subspecialties, like orthopedics).

Shit rolls downhill, huh?
Does it ever.

There are primary care physicians who now work 50- to 60-hour weeks, while there are dermatologists and plastic surgeons who work 30- to 40-hour weeks. The latter make twice as much as the former. Why?

It's not because the dermatologists or surgeons are "better doctors." It's because they are procedure-based.

A badass internist working with motivated patients can help prevent skin cancer (robbing dermatologists of some work), manage diabetes (robbing surgeons), avoid heart disease (starving interventional cardiologists), and so on. Yet, internists and family docs are some of the lowest paid physicians despite working longer weeks.

That which we pay for, we value. That which we

value, we pay for. We undervalue those preventative physicians who keep us healthy, yet overvalue those who help us when we're sick.

What does that mean for psychiatrists?

Because mental health isn't tangible or something you can drill a screw into, we're considered less valuable in the current financial system. I finished a five-year combined program (pediatrics, adult psychiatry, and child psychiatry) and was able to see and hear from both medical and mental health vantage points.

The best part of pediatrics for me was "anticipatory guidance," which is when your pediatrician teaches you what your baby is doing and what's coming down the pike. If psychiatry was afforded the same leeway, we could pre-empt a ton of prejudiced thinking to help our young patients grow up to believe that they can accomplish their dreams and be happy.

Are you saying you should be paid as much as a surgeon?

Yes and no.

I'm saying the system should let each physician build our ideal practices, charge our own rates for quality services, and let our informed and financially equipped patients be the ultimate arbiter of "what's more important."

For argument's sake, let's crunch the prerequisites:

Child Psychiatrist & General Surgeon: both finish
four years of medical school
Child Psychiatrist & General Surgeon: both finish
five-year residencies

Disclaimer: There are easy surgery programs just as
there are cush psych programs. My supposition is
based on my program where, as a Triple Board
Resident, we balanced pediatrics and psychiatry
simultaneously (thus, my strong opinions).

I would assert that a 10-hour pancreas surgery is at
least comparable to five years of regularly managing
agitation in a strong, teenage, nonverbal autistic
male.

**Well, if you get paid that kinda money, then you
better be perfect, right?**
This is one of the weirder parts of medicine.

Physicians are extremely well-trained, educated
guessers. As soon as a doctor says, "I know this with
100% certainty to be true," some new innovation or
quirk proves that doctor wrong. Doctors have done
themselves a disservice by not acknowledging this
humanism. Business-wise, it's never a good idea to
say that you're fallible (imagine Starbucks saying,
"Hey, our coffee is pretty good, but not the best").
Obviously, it wouldn't go down well. So, physicians

are kinda stuck.

We're living in a time of great change, with fallible people helping fallible people. It behooves us as doctors to lead the charge in returning to niceness and humanism. When patients recognize themselves in their physicians, we all benefit.

If doctors are kind and fallible, then why do they double-book?

It's always a money issue, nothing personal. Healthcare (which includes the art of medicine) is a service industry, and if a service isn't rendered, then no money is made. If no money is made, then the physician loses the means to practice his/her art.

Think back to our Starbucks example. Imagine that Starbucks booked five minute appointments for coffee lovers instead of their first-come, first-served queue format. What happens to their bottom line when those people who reserved a spot don't show up? The natural inclination is for that business to either decrease the time further (two minute appointments) or double book in the hopes that at least one will show up. Double-booking is purely a business decision. *(And let's not even think about those aficionados that just drop in and would have to wait to get their espressos. *shudder*)*

Some models of medical care (like urgent treatment centers) use a queue format. Others, like psychiatry practices, use a protected time model, while primary care uses a hybrid of the two.

<u>Chapter 5: Hospitals</u>

Why do most hospitals have the nicest everything?
Because the hospital is a business and that business is competing with other businesses.

Hmmm...if hospitals are businesses, why won't they list their prices?
Very good question.

When I've approached hospital administrators, their replies are the same: Chargemasters (the price guide for everything that they charge) are private proprietary documents.   For them to release them to the public means their competition (other hospitals) might undercut them.

Then whose best interest are they working toward?

Here's your first active learning assignment: Call your public hospital administrator's office (which you pay for via your taxes) and ask them that question.

Send your response to **health@togetherforward.org**, as I'd love to hear what they come up with.

Hospital administrators straddle a difficult line because their goal is to make money while showing that patient care is important. Strangely enough, the growth in the number of hospital administrators dwarfs the corresponding curve of physician growth:

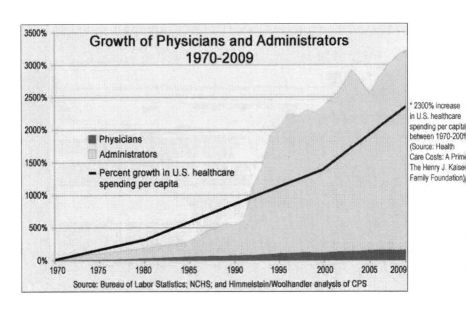

Are hospital administrative costs adding to the cost problem more than they are helping? Yup.

(Editor's Note: The same is happening in education. Be sure to check out **Forget Obama, Trump Ignored Volume 2 - EDUCATION!** *Out soon!)*

So, you hate hospital administrators?
No. I believe the hospital administration should work *for* the physicians who are in charge of the healthcare system.

Unfortunately, there are rules (some are justified) about physicians owning the hospitals they work at and refer to. Administrators (as a field) have skillsets that most physicians either lack or wish to avoid. The best way forward is for every physician to employ administrators that work towards their patient care goals and philosophy.

And what about public hospitals?
If you're going to make an ergonomic hospital, the new Parkland Hospital in Dallas, Texas is an incredible example. I've had the pleasure of treating patients there and its design is fantastic.

It also cost $1.27 billion. Why? Because no one building a company can do everything and do it well. Public hospitals serve an important purpose for managing community care, but their purview is too broad.

I would suggest public hospitals limit their scope to a few areas (e.g., major communicable diseases like TB) and leave everything else (surgeries, emergency care, and common medical admissions) to private hospitals who compete with quality and price.

But what about teaching hospitals? How will we train new doctors and nurses?
That's a discussion worth having. Turn to Chapter 13.

Chapter 6: Drug Companies

Aren't they evil, too?
No. Like health insurance companies (Chapter 2), they are private businesses looking to turn a profit.

But to charge $1,200 for an EpiPen?! That's crazy!
Not really. The EpiPen people are selling the injection delivery system, not the medicine itself. The medicine itself is hella cheap. If we all taught ourselves to give injections, we wouldn't be having this conversation.

The EpiPen people patented their nifty clicker, then cornered the market. And while our attention was elsewhere, they jacked up the price. Savvy business technique, yes, but shitty public relations and marketing.

But they have to recoup the costs of trials, research, and development, right?
Sure. I have no problem with a business creating a product and protecting their valuable intellectual property. In fact, they can continue to charge whatever they want for however long they want.

Favoring is the issue. The government, private health insurance companies, and drug manufacturers have a shadowy twisted system that protects and promotes certain drugs/companies over other drugs/companies. This perverts the few free market principles we do have.

Well, American drugs are best; I don't want stuff from overseas.
Out-of-country pharmaceutical rebranding is one of the most amazing sleights of hand because major American drug companies sell their same products overseas under a different name. They may call it something different, but the chemical structure is the same for a quarter of the price, meaning American companies are charging Americans more.

Sure, there are some chemicals used overseas that our FDA hasn't approved, but most meds are bioequivalent (i.e. they work the same way) in the French human body and the American human body.

Then why can't we get those same drugs cheaper in the states?

Because it's illegal. Read Steven Brill's *America's Bitter Pill* and try not to scream.

Chapter 7: HIPAA

Why do I have to repeat my story?
Because we're incredibly protective of our privacy.
As Americans fleeing the British monarchy,
information was power. As Americans trying to
protect our autonomy, information is power.

We enacted privacy rules to prevent stigma and to
honor that autonomy. The problem is that now the
rules are so outdated and rigid that we end up
duplicating exams and procedures because we can't
access prior records.

**But didn't you get my records from my other
doctor?**
Probably not. You would have had to sign a "release
of information," which periodically expires and if
you don't denote EXACTLY what you want
released, your old provider will err on the side of

caution and send nothing...or send the least amount to fulfill your request.

Why aren't you all on the same system?

Beats me. The VA (Chapter 12) uses the same system, so they have proven it's possible. It's clunky and old, but a veteran's records follow them everywhere they go, provided it's a VA hospital or clinic.

All patients and healthcare providers could be on one commercially available system. We simply choose not to.

Well, I want to be in full control of who knows what about me.

I agree. But I think there's a technical solution to this rather than an administrative one.

Two party authentication, physical ID tokens, biometrics—these are all creative ways to handle information access without strangling collaboration.

But what if it gets hacked?

If the recent Equifax breach has taught us anything, it's that private companies have only so much money for and expertise on cybersecurity. While no computer program is impenetrable, I'd prefer to have a commercial system housed behind the protective cyberwalls of the entire federal government. As it stands, *there are over 2,000 individual medical record systems*, all of which would have to devote time and profit to staying ahead of cyberterrorists.

<u>Chapter 8: YOU!!!</u>

What'd I do?
You forgot how to dream and you lost your creativity. Further, you also think doctors are infallible (partly our fault). You began to believe that there's such a thing as a free lunch, and that amazing things happen without any sacrifice on your part. You bought into the idea that "if it's free, gimme three," never recognizing that you're actually paying with your freedoms and liberties instead of with your hard earned cash. You over-consume and over-indulge, knowing that "the bill always comes due," yet you blame others for your current state of health.

Whoa! I'm the victim here!
No, you're not.

Seventy-five to eighty-five percent of morbidity comes from our lifestyle choices. Morbidity is essentially defined as sickness. In other words, more often than not, you cause your own illness.

Not washing your hands, eating poorly, not exercising, poor sleep, having unreasonable expectations, listening to reality TV stars about vaccines...these all lead to worsening personal and public health. I'm not asking for sainthood with healthcare choices. I'm asking that you be mindful and reasonable about health resource use.

But I have a right to be happy, don't I?
Of course you do. It's written into our Declaration of Independence.

You don't, however, have the right to make someone else pay for the results of your choices. Every parent teaches their kids some basics: use your manners, keep your hands to yourself, eat your veggies, don't play with fire, be nice to your elders. Yet, somewhere along the way, we stopped using those manners. We stopped eating our veggies. We began playing politics and trolling one another. We gave up liberty and autonomy for convenience and less pain. And then we have the audacity to expect someone to fix us. All that drama has led to this moment. Now is our time to turn the ship.

But what about my job?
Almost 10% of Americans are employed in healthcare thus many of us have a vested interest in having a system that pays well.

But it's also a perverse system that pays well in one hand while robbing you on the other. Health benefits are a large perk for all jobs in and out of the healthcare field. When we uncouple healthcare from employment, some amazing things will happen (see Chapter 10).

Chapter 9: The Shrink's Fix – Part 2

So, how the hell are you gonna roll out something like this after you've insulted everyone and pissed them off?
By doing it for the kids!

People will take care of their kids and their cars—I've witnessed this first hand as a pediatrician and child psychiatrist.

The rollout is done in five sections:

- Kids, birth to 18
- Adults with Developmental and Intellectual Disabilities & Adults with Chronic Illnesses
- Military Veterans
- Geriatrics (65+)
- Able-bodied and able-minded adults (the rest of us)

Why are kids first? They don't have jobs!
Correct. It's because they don't work (and they're our
future) that we should give them all the tools they
need to be successful adults. Stressing them out,
denying them care, feeding them junk food—we are
creating the very beasts that later feed the medico-
insurance complex.

Kids generally start off healthy, then become ill.
Genetic/metabolic conditions notwithstanding, the
majority of children require very little medical
intervention in the grand scheme of things.
Capitalizing on this with preventative care and
proactive health education means we save a ton of
money later on.

Why add the disabled next?
As a society, we've stated that kids should not work
and cannot be expected to financially contribute to
running our country.

The same is true of individuals with developmental
and intellectual disabilities and with chronic illnesses.
We know that care coordination (e.g., proactive
social work, pooling resources, and engaging
caregivers and community systems) decreases health
care costs for this cohort. Adding them in after
establishing a working pattern with our kiddos just
makes sense.

Yay for veterans!

Yay indeed. These women and men have given their bodies and souls to defend the fundamental morals and values of our country. They deserve to be taken care of.

In my plan, veterans would be treated as standard adults who still must pay for their care, but who get a nice debit card (paid for by the Department of Defense) to buy their care where they want, when they want.

And what about old folks?
As a growing demographic, people age 65+ are next in line because they've earned it. Whether I agree with their tactics or decisions, they've helped make America great (it never lost its greatness, by the way).

For older people, coordination of care is key. We get greater economies of scale when we streamline their medical care with mental health care, resource management (food, money, living), and social interaction.

We need to have a frank and candid discussion about end-of-life care because everyone will die. Ensuring the journey of life ends with dignity is a gift to both our loved ones and ourselves.

So, I'm last?
Yup. I think there's actually a well-known document that says, "the last shall be first and the first shall be last." I think that applies here.

Able-bodied and able-minded adults owe a particular debt to the very society that spawned them. Spiderman's Uncle Ben said that "with great power comes great responsibility." Being able to wake up, go to work, provide for yourself and family, and sleep soundly is a great power. Treating others as you'd like to be treated means that we all win.

Why'd you make it state-based?

I'm going to make an assumption that people in your state know your needs better than people in a different state. When you create a state-based system, adjustments can be made faster and there is more direct accountability for health decisions.

Secondly, in this plan state governments work directly with the State Health Company Board of Directors to mitigate taxes and ensure that the General Health Fee is commensurate to the cost of living, unemployment rates, wage growth, and other financial markers.

Thirdly, a system at the state level creates another layer of competition. If certain states have competitive services that other states don't have, losing business provides an incentive for the lagging states to get their acts together (or people will leave/move).

Fourthly, as a private company (and not an extension of the government), a State Health

Company will be more administratively manageable compared to a national private company.

Lastly, state-based systems allow federal workers to concentrate on other concerns (defense, immigration, fiscal policy) without grinding everyday life to a halt every time a Congressman pitches a fit about healthcare.

Argh. I'm still having a tough time conceptualizing this.
Think of it like Costco.

Everyone pays a membership fee. Inside Costco is a plethora of items and services you can buy (they're not free). Items in the same field compete for your business through quality and price (like Brawny vs. Bounty). And because Costco buys products in bulk, they pass those savings on to you.

My idea works similarly. You pay a membership fee, which gains you access to items and services that you buy but you'll know the costs before you do. Items and services in the same field compete for your business through quality, price, and service. And because you've paid your membership, you're entitled to medication discounts since your State Health Company buys medications in bulk.

Now overlay that idea with municipal water companies. Everyone pays a base rate, whereafter you pay for what you use. There are always "free" water resources in a community for those who are struggling, but those "free" resources are subsidized by private entities (like restaurants, city hall, private residences, etc.)

So, if I hear you correctly, we pay a fee, right?
Yes. Everyone must pay something because that which you don't pay for, you don't value.

Chapter 10: Results

Higher Wages

When companies can no longer imprison you in the job you hate with the lure of health benefits, what will they do to keep you from exiting stage right?

You guessed it, dear reader. They'll pay you more.

Or they won't, and you can leave and go to the competitor who will recognize your value and pay you more.

Either way, your wages will go up because businesses can now afford to do so, since they do not have to shoulder the cost of your medical care.

Patient Choice

A la carte pricing will pave the way to patient choice. All physicians, nurses, therapists, and the like will post their prices, and you, being the savvy shopper you are, get to choose. Allopathic, osteopathic, naturopathic, chiropractic—visit the providers who resonate with you.

Caution: Beware social rating sites for medical quality because each private interaction is private for a reason. What you read online is often only one side, so take it with a grain of salt.

Physician Autonomy
Physicians are the CEOs of their skill and practice. Sure, some may join groups, but in the Internet age, you'll see integration and convenience improve as physicians compete to improve your care.

Lower Prices Through Transparency
Transparency is great because it decreases prices while increasing quality. With no more hidden chargemasters, you'll have clear lists of costs so that you'll always know what you're responsible for paying.

Economic Growth
Better employee pay. Higher business operating budgets. More spending. More purposeful consumption. We all win!

Citizenship Neutral
Just as anyone with an address and the money for the fee can buy a Costco membership, joining the state-based private health company means everyone gets access to high-quality, affordable healthcare.

Undocumented individuals won't be able to choose Board members, but that wouldn't keep them from purchasing their care directly (just like the rest of us).

Mental Health Parity

Medicare skewed medical value when it reimbursed procedures more than non-procedures (see Chapter Four). With that stipulation removed, we'll now place quality mental health care alongside quality medical and surgical services. Offered yearly as part of the standard visit, seeing a psychiatrist will be as common as seeing your dentist. This will end mental health stigma completely.

Respectful of Women's Health

Whether you're pro-choice or anti-choice (because really, who's "anti-life?"), we all agree that managing decisions during pregnancy isn't easy. Whether to carry to term, what meds to be on, or evaluating risk exposure, all of these factors are private decisions.

Changing healthcare finance allows private decisions to stay private because patients will have the financial ability to see the health providers of their choice and pay them directly (patients can always elect not to have the provider submit the code for reimbursement).

Veteran Support

Our VA system is broken and weird. Why we make veterans drive hours to get care when there are physicians in their own town is baffling. This new system gives veterans the opportunity to see a physician near them, and to choose the ancillary services that complement a solid medical treatment plan.

Individual Accountability
No one should pay for my love of Whataburger Patty Melts. Only I am responsible for the metabolic consequences of delicious meat, cheese, and spices with tender onions on buttered Texas toast.

People value what they pay for and pay for what they value. When everyone has skin in the healthcare game, they have a vested interest in keeping costs down by staying healthy because it keeps money in their pockets.

Federal Government Efficiency
Imagine what happens when there's less on senators' plates to deal with.

I often wonder if Congress creates problems for them to solve, so taking healthcare off their agenda gives them time and energy to focus on other big items like a nuclear North Korea, immigration, cybersecurity, climate change, and national infrastructure (including national broadband Internet.)

Increased Individual Liberty

It is our constitutional right to make dumb choices if they don't negatively impact the rights of others. These civil liberties drive innovations in service and spawn entirely new industries.

Local Accountability
It's humbling to provide a service to someone then have them in turn hand you their hard earned money. The patient-physician bond is already strong, but adding a financial layer takes the fiduciary responsibility even further.

Direct care creates local accountability and builds stronger social networks.

Increased Civic Engagement
Holding politicians accountable (every two to six years) is hard. Gerrymandering and politicking make it almost impossible to get irresponsible politicians out the door.

With the private board overseeing the State Health Company, the directors are directly accountable to state citizens who can recall them whenever they choose (per company bylaws).

Medical Bankruptcy
This will now be a thing of the past. People will be able to budget and plan for medical catastrophes so the cost of care doesn't wipe out their personal bank accounts. And remember: Your state Health Fund

reimburses for costs unrelated to lifestyle choices, so the rest you can cover with catastrophic insurance.

Improved Social Mobility

Imagine leaving a state where the jobs are scarce so you can move somewhere new knowing that the healthcare provided there is transparent and accessible. Uncoupling healthcare from your employer means you can find new employment in places that resonate with you and your family.

Chapter 11: "The Won't Works"

Single Payer

Imagine you trained passionately to master your craft for 11 years nonstop. Imagine that you missed births, deaths, weddings, and funerals for those you love in order to learn that craft. Imagine that you take thousands of dollars' worth of tests and insure yourself for thousands of more dollars. Now imagine you finally open your business to showcase your skill only to discover that someone without your ability or training looks you in the eye and says, "You can't do that."

A single-payer system means that some entity (likely the government) will employ legions of non-physicians to render decisions on care for patients. **Would you go for that?**

Most physicians wouldn't either. There will be senators touting that the administrative costs for Medicare are lower than private commercial insurers, and they are correct. But there are more transparent ways of decreasing costs than inserting an unnecessary middleman. I work directly with my patients to find what's best for them and their situation; for anyone (physician or not) to tell me otherwise is a non-starter.

Physicians treat patients because they love helping people feel better. But make no mistake: They are incredibly protective of their autonomy and having a singular agency dictating to us what we can and cannot do is akin to a turd in the punchbowl.

ACA/AHCA/BCRA/OC

Don't waste your time looking up what these abbreviations mean. They're all synonymous with a financial system built on commercial insurance companies. Since they each answer to their respective boards and shareholders (not you, the citizen), patient care is secondary to profit.

Commercial insurance premiums will only increase. Forever. Because they can. We can build processes on top of this broken system (like reinsurance in Chapter 2), or we can scrap it all together. I vote for the latter.

Free Market

A completely free market system won't work in healthcare and would actually lead to a worsening of health finance disparity. The rich would only be seen by the rich, and the rest of us would have to fend for ourselves.

That's why I like a "hybrid" system that provides
basic preventative care, layers on coverage for health
events that are unrelated to your lifestyle choices,
and then gives individuals responsibility for the rest.

Chapter 12: The VA – A Case Study of Single Payer

Isn't the VA wonderful?
In theory, yes.

In execution, nope.

As a government-run and funded system, the bureaucracy is intense and waste is extreme. Simple procedures turn into complicated odysseys. The VA system is the innovative opposite of how our country runs. Here's your next active learning assignment: Talk with a veteran who must use the VA system. Ask them what they like and don't like. Ask them how far they travel for care, and if the VA is responsive to their needs/requests. I think you'll see a pattern.

But it's a model for integrated care, right?
Correct. And that's one of its biggest downfalls, because it's hard to be everything to everyone. When

I worked at the VA as a psychiatry resident, there'd be common medical conditions psychiatrists wanted to manage (e.g,. diabetes or high blood pressure) but we couldn't because we weren't primary care providers.

Don't our veterans deserve the best?
Yes, which is why they should have the choice to go where they want for care. Competition improves quality, but the VA has no competition since it's a closed system.

What happens to the VA in your diabolical plan?
It becomes just like every other private hospital, but will be run by physicians who specialize in veteran-centered care, and who work diligently to recruit and retain veterans as patients through innovative medical practices and targeted marketing.

Chapter 13: Odds and Ends, Questions and Concerns

You know nonprofits don't have shareholders, right?

Yes, astute reader. I'm banking on this book starting a conversation and, subsequently, a different tax category [e.g., 501(c)(3), 501(c)(4), etc]. For this to work best, each person needs a vested equal stake in the State Health Company so that it eliminates perverse incentives (i.e. you won't exploit your customer because YOU are the customer).

"Personal lifestyle choices"? That's a slippery slope. How will you parse these details?

Full disclosure: Full discussion of this concept requires national discussion. I don't presume to be able to nuance the details in this e-book, and it'd be the height of hubris for me to say I can address every concern for every situation.

In general, the "tie goes to the runner" so when in doubt, the General Health Fund will pay for care. But luckily, we've built an entire system of risk scores for everything: age, gender, genes, diet, exercise, sleep, drug use, and careers. We have established guides that guess the percentage effects of lifestyle choices on the creation and maintenance of every illness I can think of. Our state health companies would then use these to set their chargemaster rates.

Ugh. What if I don't want to pay the General Health Fee or pay into the State General Health Fund?

You don't have to. That's the beauty of the plan; it's 100% voluntary. However, opting out means you won't have access to the universal electronic medical record and you won't have the financial leverage to bring drug costs down.

So, what would happen to me if I decided to opt out entirely? Break it down for me.

You'd basically continue to use the old system. You'd see a physician and your records would be local (not in the universal electronic medical record). You'd pay them directly and if you needed medications or labs, you'd pay the retail price (without the State Health Company bulk discount). Thus, you can live a full and present life without buying into your state health system.

And if doctors don't want to participate in the program? What then?
All physician practices will essentially be private businesses. They will post whatever price they'd like for the services they render. Patients would pay them directly and when the physician codes the action in the universal electronic medical record, the state reads the code and sends the patient a reimbursement depending on the money value tied to the code.

For example, if I charged $100 for an annual physical and the state chargemaster covers $50, you'd pay me $100, I evaluate you and submit the code. You then get $50 pulled from the General Health Fund and sent to your bank account.

Why do preventative visits only provide medications for three months?
I made it up. Three months is a nice period of time to monitor for progress (which is why most companies have quarterly meetings) but each state will decide the best amount of time for its populace.

Concierge? Direct Pay? Why so many names?
Because all doctors are different. The realm of medicine is broad and has three basic branches: medical, surgical, and mental health. Each branch requires its own "ideal practice" model, and what's good for one might not work for the other.

For example, a "concierge" model typically means

69

paying a fee and then being able to access your doctor as often as you want. For my practice (psychiatry), this actually goes against my treatment philosophy since I encourage my patients to work through their concerns using the skills they've learned with me, rather than by coming back to my office as often as they like.

So, which medical model is best?
I suggest that because they are all physician-led, all of them are viable under my plan.

What happens to health insurance?
It will still exist, you just won't "need" it, and it will become what it was intended to be: catastrophic coverage for medical catastrophes.

Insurance at its most basic is you betting against yourself that something will or will not happen. Car insurance is betting that you won't get into an accident, and there are tables of data to show your risk. While I'm not a psychic, I know you have a 100% chance of needing healthcare this year. So, why buy insurance against a 100% risk? Why not just pay for it directly when you need it?

What role will Congress have in your plan?
The federal government won't be involved in your healthcare AT ALL. No more reliance on Congress to pass a budget. Bye reconciliation! (whatever "reconciliation" means...)

Don't you need a proof of concept?

I have one. Without taking insurance, my private practice was able to generate over $200,000 last year (of course, running a small business eats all that up, but that's the American dream, right?). There are direct-pay family medicine clinics, surgery clinics, and dermatology practices all across the country that prove this idea works.

But that's only for rich people, right?

Nope. I have patients of all backgrounds who pay out-of-pocket. In turn, I make sure to deliver high quality and convenient care to them, as I believe in being a good steward of their time and finances. Though, I would say it's only for "motivated people." Being mindful of your health, purposeful in your decisions, and intentional in your thoughts takes work. Our current health finance system breeds laziness, whereas the new model encourages education and accountability.

How would you fund medical schools?

My first thought is that doctors should provide that type of apprenticeship for their fellow up-and-coming docs. Medical school is, unfortunately, caught up in the over-inflated pricing scheme of higher education (that'll be my next book). Nursing, pharmacy, and allied health, among others, would all be funded by their respective professions, as well.

How would you fund medical research?

The standard ways: taxes, educational institutions, and private companies. In this way, Americans will have money in their pockets to directly invest in bench research (www.experiment.com).

What happens to health co-ops?

I think co-ops are awesome because they are part of such an intentional act. You're promising to pool money and pay attention to what you eat, drink, and do, which minimizes risk and saves you money. I believe co-ops will blossom under my idea.

How will we have "educated citizens" to make good health choices when our public schools are struggling?

The education reform ideas in "Save Yo' Self: Volume 2 – how to fix education" will be paid for by the health savings from healthcare reform. So, let's tackle this beast first.

How do we ensure physicians do the right thing and not price gouge?

Each state has a governmental medical board that regulates the licensing and reprimanding of their physicians. Every patient will continue to have this avenue as a means to file grievances related to standards of care. Price gouging will fall under the same rules as general business laws within specific states.

Chapter 14: Grand Compromises

What does compromise have to do with this?
The best compromise makes everyone feel like
they're losing. So, let's get started pissing people off.

Allow nurse practitioners to be unsupervised
The idea of "mid-level providers," like nurse
practitioners (NPs) and physician assistants (PAs),
fits into the narrative that we have a "shortage" of
medical providers. I don't believe there's a shortage;
I think there are geographic and financial
inefficiencies that are best addressed by physician-led
teams. For states that feel it's necessary to allow NPs
and PAs to practice without supervision, I say "bring
it."

I know and respect some amazing nurse
practitioners who are great at their jobs *because* they
know their limits. A few of them live in states where
they can practice independently and still choose to

keep a close supervisory relationship with a physician because they see patient safety as paramount.

There are strong physician forces advocating for mandatory supervision of nurse practitioners, but I think "mandatory" breeds animosity. Instead, I believe we should let NPs practice their brand of nursing while ensuring they have higher malpractice rates, commensurate to their hours of training. NPs have only 10% of the clinical training hours (2,000 hours) of a physician (20,000 hours), so it seems reasonable for their rates to be 90% higher than their physician counterparts. For unsupervised NPs to have lower malpractice rates (the current arrangement) suggests their brand of nursing is less risky than physician-led medicine. Alternatively, NPs who have quality supervising agreements with physicians could, in turn, have lower malpractice rates.

Create "medical hospitality" and expand home health to create competition and lower cost

At its most basic definition, what is a hospital?

It's a building with rooms for rent where a person stays for a period of time and receives personal interaction from a medical professional. We've proven that home health works; who's to say this can't happen in a hotel environment?

Enter "medical hospitality." Imagine how hospital

prices will fall when people can get their doctor or home health aide to stop by their hotel to do rounds. Imagine being able to have family stay next door to keep you company while you rehab.

Yes, there are obviously some logistics to work out, like biohazard disposal for a hotel, but the component parts to create hospital competition already exist.

Remove 501(c)(3) tax exemptions for all hospitals and churches

Despite growing up in a Pentecostal household and attending the biggest Baptist university in the world, I never really understood the justification for church tax-exemption, especially since these buildings are generally well air-conditioned, use lots of energy, and take up residential/commercial space we could use for other reasons.

I find the same is true of hospitals. They are businesses designed to make money, so I'm not sure why any of them would get a tax exemption.

I define charity care as any care rendered that incurs a fee that the patient can't pay. I'd suggest that churches and hospitals have their 501(c)(3) tax designation removed and, for every dollar they spend in charity care, they can then write that off as a tax deduction.

Charity care means hospitals and churches, rather than the government, would pay the General Health Fee for those that can't afford it. After all, isn't that what those entities exist to do?

Allow physicians to own hospitals
Who knows best how to manage your household? You do.

As Americans, we've established that the head of household comes with certain rights and privileges. When people come into your home, you might offer the fancy flavored bubble water or something straight from the tap.

As physicians, we know how to create environments that heal and nurture. Allowing physicians to own buildings of healing means they are ultimately responsible for the patient experience. If they fail, they go out of business.

Allow telemedicine across all states
Professionally, I don't care to provide telemedicine. I did it during my training in residency, and it didn't click with my personality or style. But telemedicine is helpful for many, and my personal preferences shouldn't taint the research that shows it improves access to care.

Currently, telemedicine is regulated at the state level because physicians are regulated at the state level. I don't suggest we change the state regulatory board model, but a national telemedicine plan that allows us to cross state borders is worth discussing.

Enforce mandatory participation by all health-related providers and State Board of Directors with the Sunshine Act

Every patient deserves to know who their providers are talking to. The "Sunshine Act" is a program to increase transparency of financial relationships that your medical provider may have. Research shows that marketing by drug and medical equipment companies make a difference in the clinical decisions that health providers make (dentists, doctors, nurses, and therapists).

<u>Chapter 15: Residency</u>

Is residency as awesome as on TV?
It's better. Being able to learn patient care is an
honor and a privilege. While TV makes residency
look dramatic, real medicine is not very sexy. It's
thrilling to diagnose a rare disease or participate in
an exciting procedure, the long hours but, the stress
on family, friends, and body are less than awesome.

How do residents get paid?
This is a black hole in our understanding. Residency
programs are controlled by the Accreditation
Council for Graduate Medical Education. It's a
nonprofit made up of the American Board of
Medical Specialties (ABMS), American Hospital
Association (AHA), American Medical Association

(AMA), Association of American Medical Colleges (AAMC), Council of Medical Specialty Societies, American Osteopathic Association (AOA), and American Association of Colleges of Osteopathic Medicine (AACOM). The ACGME essentially makes sure that residencies are legit so that physicians have a standard and don't become one of the "snake oil" salesmen that were once rampant.

Ahem. How do residents get paid?

Whoops, sorry. Residency funding is a mix of government funds (set by the Centers for Medicare & Medicaid Services or CMS), the host hospital, and the host university. The exact mix of who pays what is a highly guarded secret; all residents know is that once a month they get a salary, and they work upward of 80 hours a week for 3 to 7 years.

What's keeping residents from being active in health reform?

Two things: workload and perspective. Residents are consuming massive amounts of information and learning to become the head of a medical team. Regardless of whether that team is a singular person (solo practice) or a large group, each physician is charged with expertise in his or her area. There's very little time to organize and fight against health economic forces.

Couple that with lack of transparency about how residency is funded and how their future selves actually make money, and you have a clinically knowledgeable workforce with large knowledge gaps in health finance and avenues for reform.

Chapter 16: Nurse Practitioners

What is a nurse practitioner?
Nurse practitioners are registered nurses (RNs) who complete master's courses that combine nursing practice and nursing theory with some of the basics of medical diagnosis.

Do doctors have beef with nurse practitioners?
As people, of course not. They are men and women who want to help others feel better, which is exactly why physicians practice medicine. However, professionally, their very existence bends the law, blurs lines, and costs the system more money.

The practice of medicine is defined as the privilege of diagnosing a condition and guiding treatment. Each state has delegated the "practice of medicine" as the exclusive right of physicians. A physician is defined as someone who completes medical school and then completes another 1 year of "on-the-job" training. Only then (and after lots of money and paperwork) are you allowed to "practice" medicine and only for each state where you've applied.

How do nurse practitioners bend the law?
Because they are practicing medicine without a medical license. Remember, a medical license can only be obtained by going to medical school. There is a push by some nurse practitioners to clarify that they're not practicing medicine but are instead practicing "advanced practice nursing."

Gotcha. So how is advanced practice nursing different than medicine?
That's where it gets very sticky. Remember, if diagnosing and guiding treatment are the sole lawful privilege of physicians, allowing any other profession to diagnose and guide treatment is unlawful. Currently, "advanced practice nursing" includes diagnosing and guiding treatment so you can see how the lines are blurry.

Then what are 300,000 nurse practitioners doing?
Good question and one that you deserve to hear

directly from them. As a profession, it's their responsibility to ensure they are abiding by the laws and to explain to patients who they are and what their scope is. Unfortunately, because of the way health finance works, physicians are stuck doing "quick visits," which creates the "shortage." There are a slew of entrepreneurial nurse practitioners who have found an opening to help patients (good) at the expense of transparency (bad). For example, there now exists the designation "DNP," which stands for doctorate in nursing practice, and those individuals call themselves "Dr."

Wait. I'm confused. How would I know if I'm seeing a medical doctor or a doctor of nursing practice?
You won't – unless you're paying attention to the badge and how they introduce themselves. Unfortunately, there are lots of individuals with DNPs who aren't forthcoming with their credentials and training. Thus, you may be seeing someone with 10% of a physician's training and not know it.

What's the difference between a nurse practitioner and a physician assistant?

Physician assistants are trained for 2,000 hours in the medical model during their graduate school training. They are knowledgeable about how to diagnose and treat, but they cannot do so independently of physicians. Physician assistants are under the close eye of their state's medical board.

Nurse practitioners are nurses trained in the nursing model. Thus, they aren't taught how to diagnose and treat at the beginning of their training. Nurse practitioner graduate school is a 500-1,500 hour "crash course" in diagnosing and treatment ... err ... advanced nurse practice. (See how confusing this is?) Nurse practitioners are under the purview of their state's nursing board.

So you're saying they should go to PA school?
We live in a free country; they can do whatever they're legally able to do. Completing a PA program will ensure that all physician extenders (or midlevel providers) have a solid medical foundation on which to make medical decisions under the oversight of a physician.

You've been advocating that physician assistants and nurse practitioners pay higher malpractice rates. Why?

Malpractice is determined partly on your risk for patient harm. Recognizing that no one goes into healthcare to actively harm people, sometimes errors occur. If patients are harmed due to our negligence, they deserve to be compensated for that. Physician malpractice rates are set based on geographic location and specialty.

Well, I like my nurse practitioner more than my physician, and I want to keep seeing them.
By all means, do so. We live in the greatest country in the world, and it's your right to seek health advice from whomever you wish. I only advocate for transparency and fairness. You should know you're seeing a nurse practitioner and should know exactly how many clinical hours of training they've had. Additionally, they should be required to hold malpractice rates and insurance policies commiserate to their risk and level of training.

How can we fix the "nurses practicing medicine" thing?
One idea is for all nurse practitioners to complete physician assistant training since the PA profession is legally practicing medicine under the purview of a licensed physician.

Let me get this straight. Doctors created nurse practitioners, and now you want to eliminate them?
Is it coincidental that Medicare was established in 1965 at the same time the first nurse practitioner program was created? Medicare is now an outdated and flawed health finance system. With the creation of the internet, telepresence, and point-of-care technology, physicians and physician assistants (when their practices are structured correctly) can more than meet the demand for medical care without adding confusion about roles. Add in incentives for people to prevent illness and this decreases the pool of people needing medical care. (Chapter Eight)

What happens to bedside nursing?
That's the great unknown. There has been a shortage of bedside nurses for years, and their ranks and that shortage is slated to grow. With the explosion of NP programs (some of which are completely online), more bedside nurses are opting for this training, which takes them out of direct patient care and puts them in the "in-between." Working "in-between" means that there are less direct care nurses in

hospitals and clinics and more non-physicians in the medical space. It's quite a pickle.

Chapter 17: Medicare and HSAs

"I like my Medicare. I want to keep it."
During my book signings and presentations on
reforming health finance, I heard this sentiment
from older patrons who were very concerned that I
was advocating for elimination of a social program
they've paid into. Here's the key: Your money is your
money. Instead, I advocate transitioning all of your
contributions to date into a health spending account
(HSA) that you can use for any medical, health,
mental health, dental, or vision costs.

**But how will that be enough money? Healthcare
is so expensive!**
Once Chapter One is created, transitioning the
Medicare system into a lifetime HSA will further
stretch your healthcare dollar.

What if I want Medicare to stay exactly the

same?

I'd say that you're fighting a losing battle. Medicare enshrines a layer of administration between you and your physician. At some point, when physicians tire of being told what they can and cannot do by Medicare administrators, they will "opt out" of Medicare, thereby decreasing the number of physicians in the network. The result: You'll be locked into a system that has no physicians, thereby increasing wait time and frustration.

Then we should link Medicare to state licensure. That'll force doctors to be part of the system and accept Medicare patients.

Liberty is a central tenet of American society. To force a physician into a system that jeopardizes his or her ability to make a living for his or her family is a step too far. A much more appropriate step is to ensure patients have the funds to buy their care and let physicians compete for your healthcare dollars.

Chapter 18: Physician Suicide & Substance Abuse

Why are physicians killing themselves?
Physicians are humans, with all the joys and heartaches that every other human endures. Unique expectations are placed on physicians (never be wrong, see as many people as possible, document everything, click "this" box, etc.). These expectations collide with our own savior complex (stand strong, stay until the job is done, exhaust all options, etc.) in a deadly fashion.

How many physicians commit suicide each year?
Strangely enough, we don't track this data. One passionate physician, Pamela Wible, MD, has personally taken on documenting physician suicide as a calling, but she can only do so much. There are

an estimated 800,000 physicians in America, and we guess that about 400 take their lives each year (50 per 100,000.) Compared to suicide in the general population (13 per 100,000), physicians are almost 4 times as likely to die from suicide. Suicide is preventable; we need to ensure each physician (like every patient) is well cared for.

And substance use?
The rates of substance use (caffeine, tobacco, alcohol, sedatives) is high. Physicians are just as prone to poor coping skills as non-physicians. Unfortunately, rather than tackle physician substance use with compassion, many state boards (who are responsible for regulating and licensing physicians) take an almost combative approach to addressing substance use in physicians. The result: underreporting by physicians and physician colleagues for fear of retribution. Imagine spending 13 years in training, driving drunk, and losing the ability to provide for yourself after 1 night of poor judgment.

You mentioned abuse. How can someone in a position of power be abused?
Employed physicians are often not in charge of the system they work for. The result: They are beholden

to all the shenanigans systems create to establish corporate pecking order. Sham peer reviews, labeling physicians as "disruptive," and 360-degree evaluations collude to denigrate the profession of medicine. Adding in the unhelpful documentation requirements of the health finance system (MACRA, MIPS, Meaningful Use) leads to bullied physicians who are burned out.

So why don't they just quit like you did?
Because they're afraid. Just like I was afraid. When I took the leap from employed to private practice, I had no idea what I was doing. I was fortunate to be single and childless; I cut my expenses and had ample financial room to make lots of mistakes. And I did. There were times in the first 3 years where I went without paying myself and had to live off my credit cards for the first time in years. Not every physician has the luxury of learning private practice like I did – at least not yet.

How does private practice fix physician suicide and abuse?
It doesn't. My point is that autonomy decreases suicide and abuse. When you feel in control of your life, your finances, and your future, you're invested in the outcome. Working with physician grassroots

groups to create physician CEO programs means that physicians can now build autonomous practices that they completely control. On the backend, Chapter One describes how to structure health finance so that patients have the funds to buy their care directly from physician CEOs. It's a win-win.

Why can't doctors get their act together?
We're working on it: www.PhysiciansRise.com

Chapter 19: Amazon, Berkshire-Hathaway, Chase, and More: The ABCs of Diversion

Yay! Healthcare is saved! Bezos, Buffet, and Dimon are coming to save the day!

Not quite. Adding trillion-dollar corporate players into a field based on two parties (patient and physician) only exacerbates the issue because the single most important issue is that patients don't have the *funds* to access care. If these men wanted to actually be helpful, they'd pay their employees more so that employees/patients could buy their care directly from physicians. Plain and simple.

But technology will help care be delivered faster and more efficiently. Right?

I believe that telemedicine and point-of-care tech

resources have a place in healthcare. However, we forget that healthcare (different than business and IT) is an intimate human interaction that's almost always best addressed in person, looking eye to eye. Transporting patients via medical Uber or creating minute clinics doesn't change the fact that humans (especially Americans) feel better when they've established a relationship with their health adviser.

Chapter 20: Aetna, Blue Cross/Blue Shield, Cigna, and More: The ABCs of Obfuscation

Things have changed a lot with health insurers since your idea launched.

Indeed! CVS/Caremark merged with Aetna, UnitedHealthcare merged with Optum and Davita, Cigna merged with ExpressScripts, and the list goes on and on. One universal theme between all these entities is obfuscation.

What is obfuscation?

Wikipedia's entry: *"Obfuscation is the obscuring of the intended meaning of communication by making the message difficult to understand, usually with confusing and ambiguous language. The obfuscation might be either unintentional or intentional (although intent usually is connoted), and is*

*accomplished with circumlocution (talking around the subject),
the use of jargon (technical language of a profession), and the
use of an argot (ingroup language) of limited communicative
value to outsiders."*
(https://en.wikipedia.org/wiki/Obfuscation)

Let's break it down in detail:
"Health insurance" has nothing to do with health
other than these companies want you to think it
does. They purposefully confuse "health coverage"
with "access to care" because they don't want to
admit that they're actively limiting your access to
care by actively limiting how much they're willing to
help you pay for it.

"Explanation of benefits" doesn't explain benefits.
It's doublespeak for, "We're drawing this process out
in hopes that you'll quit asking and we can keep your
premiums."

"Value based care" doesn't describe care's value. It
describes a payment model that punishes caregivers
for poor outcomes, even when it's due to patient
choices.

What benefit does obfuscation get them?
Confusion. As Desiderius Erasmus said, "In the land

of the blind, the one-eyed man is king." Health insurance companies have done an amazing job with intention confusion, so much so that many believe they will die or be at higher risk of dying simply because they don't have a health insurance policy. This fear drives consumption and health insurance companies are there to relieve that angst, for a monthly premium.

I thought you respected healthcare companies as businesses?
I sorta do. But seeing these huge mergers means one thing: They're after profits and not patient care. Notice that despite these new pairings of health insurance companies, pharmacies, and pharmacy benefit managers, costs STILL aren't going down?

Chapter 21: Pharmacists and Pharmacies

My pharmacist is awesome! What do they have to do with health reform?

Pharmacists are trained scientists who are experts in dispensing and the effects of medications. Occupational law prohibits pharmacists from diagnosing medical concerns but they work hand-in-hand with your physician to build a powerful treatment team. Unfortunately, they're under "gag-orders" that prevent them from telling you about cheaper medicines.

What?! That should be illegal.

Agreed. There are actually pending legislation in some states to remove this clause that's written into the contracts between pharmacies and the pharmacists that they hire. Independent pharmacists (pharmacies owned directly by an entrepreneurial pharmacist) don't often have those restrictions. They work doubly hard to get you the best price because they want you to continue to become a repeat customer.

If that's the worst of their contributions...

Not so fast. Pharmacists get bullied as much as physicians but their bullies take the form of PBM or "pharmacy benefit managers." These secret companies negotiate between your health insurance company and the pharmacy and take their cut from "administering" contracts between the two. The result: higher costs for you.

How do we fight this?

Remember obfuscation. These systems are purposefully hidden to leach money out of an already bloated health finance system. Fighting the PBM system is so difficult that I'd recommend skipping it altogether and instead, change the pharmacy free market at its very foundation (see Chapter One, *Step Six*).

Chapter 22: Money Talks

You were quoted during a lecture saying, "We can unleash trillions of dollars of economic power." How'd you come up with that number?
Like any good economist, I made it up. In all seriousness, though, imagine the economic power of thousands of new entrepreneurs in the home health, micro-hospital, and "medical hospitality" space. Imagine the surge of allied health professionals (acupuncturists, physical therapists, yogis) and mental health professionals (psychologists, therapists, counselors) who can hang a shingle and sustain vibrant practices directly with the clients they serve.

Wait a second; you're describing an economic renaissance.
Yes. When thousands of smaller companies can now compete against the CVS/Aetnas, the Amazons and

Googles, we all benefit. The answer to energy independence already exists. The solution to food security sits on a few people's hard drives. Yet you would never know it because the very thing we think is helping (the corporatization of everything) actually hinders creativity and economic growth.

When we've decoupled "health benefits" from employment and infused hundreds of millions of Americans with cash and autonomy, we'll enter the next medical renaissance.

<u>Conclusion</u>

When reasonable Americans are given reasonable options, they make reasonable choices. We live in a health finance system that favors the rich and corporate and punishes the rest of us. I do not advocate for "free care," as I recognize Americans that value having skin in the game.

There's a reason Costco members and Costco employees are happy: Transparency. Each group knows exactly what they're getting into when they join the company. We can't directly beat Medicare, Medicaid, BlueCross, Cigna, Aetna, United Healthcare, Molina, or any of the rest. Instead, let's concentrate on changing the very market forces on which they rest to favor the individual citizen. We'll win every time.

The first and most important step is to commit to fixing healthcare. Then talk about your commitment with your family, friends, neighbors, co-workers, and employers. Make it public that you aren't happy. You *aren't* satisfied. Demand better. See your therapist. Commit to personally doing better and you'll see the better all around you.

Call to Action

o Take a deep breath, and then another. You got this.

o Tell your governor to encourage statewide discussion on incorporating a State Health Company.

o Compel your governor to collaborate with other governors to adopt the PSYCH infrastructure and agreements, and to elect a Board of Directors for your state-based health company.

o Convince your Congresspeople (House and Senate) to repeal the ACA and Medicare and Medicaid Acts, along with 501(c)(3) tax designations for churches and hospitals. If they won't budge, vote in new Congresspeople who will.

o Encourage your state regulators to write new policies for medical hospitality and review telemedicine regulations, as well as change rules regarding physician-hospital ownership.

o Share the link www.changehealth.today with everyone you can think of. It's time to get the conversation started!

o Donate to Together Forward (http://www.togetherforward.org) so that we can start working on education reform next (http://www.changedu.today).

o Recycle, reduce, reuse. Walk outside for 30 minutes every day in a greenspace.

o Be kind to yourself.

End Notes

America's Bitter Pill: Money, Politics, Backroom
Deals, and the Fight to Fix Our Broken Healthcare
System by Steven Brill. 2015.

Centers for Disease Control. Power of Prevention,
2009.
https://www.cdc.gov/chronicdisease/pdf/2009-
power-of-prevention.pdf

ChangEDU Today: www.changedu.today

Change Health Today: www.changehealth.today

The Constitution of the United States of America:
https://www.archives.gov/founding-
docs/constitution-transcript

Crowdfunding Science: www.experiment.com

Ensuring America's Health: The Public Creation of
the Corporate Health Care System by Christy Ford
Chapin. 2015.

Growth of Physicians and Administrators 1970 –
2009: https://fee.org/articles/the-chart-that-could-
undo-the-us-healthcare-system/

New Parkland Memorial Hospital $16 Million Over
Budget:
https://www.dallasnews.com/news/news/2013/05
/07/new-parkland-memorial-hospital-16-million-
over-budget

Physician Financial Transparency Reports (Sunshine
Act)
https://www.ama-assn.org/practice-
management/physician-financial-transparency-
reports-sunshine-act

Progressive Psychiatry, P.A.:
www.progressivepsychiatry.org

Together Forward: www.togetherforward.org

Made in the USA
San Bernardino, CA
29 May 2018